Mango recipes for the entire family to enjoy

Delicious Mango Creations

Anita collins

Contents

DISCLAIMER

This book is as accurate and complete as possible. There may be typographical errors or mistakes in the content. This book also contains information that is only current as of the publication date. This Book is not the definitive source of information and should only be used as a guide. The book's sole purpose is to teach. The publisher or author does not guarantee the eBook's accuracy. They are not responsible for any error, omissions, or misinformation

Introduction

We'd like to take this opportunity to welcome you to the wondrous world of mango dishes, which is sure to capture the taste buds of everyone in your family. These dishes guarantee a gastronomic adventure that is not only delectable but also gratifying as a result of their abundance of vivacious flavors as well as the exotic essence of juicy mangoes. Our range of mango-infused concoctions includes everything from reviving beverages to delectable sweets and savory pleasures, and it is designed to appeal to a wide variety of taste preferences.

Mangoes, which are commonly referred to as the "king of fruits," give a touch of sweetness and lusciousness to a wide variety of recipes, giving your family's mealtimes a tropical feel as a result. It doesn't matter if you're a seasoned chef or a home cook eager to explore new culinary horizons; these recipes offer the ideal balance of simplicity and elegance, which makes them approachable and pleasant for people of all levels of cooking experience.

Choosing the Perfect Mango

Tips on selecting ripe and flavorful mangoes for your recipes.

Qualities of a Fresh Mango

Fresh mangoes possess several qualities that indicate their freshness and overall quality. Here are the key qualities to look for in a fresh mango:

Firmness:

When you give a fresh mango a little squeeze, it should have a solid consistency. It should not have a consistency that is too soft or mushy because this might be an indication of over-ripeness or rot.

Aroma:

When a mango is mature, the stem end of the fruit gives out a scent that is both sweet and delicious. Check if it has a good aroma by giving it a sniff close to the stem.

Mangoes that smell off or nasty should be avoided.

Color:

The hue of a fresh mango might vary depending on the type of mango it is. On the other hand, in general, a fresh mango will have a color that is brilliant and uniform throughout the fruit. Depending on the kind, its color can range anywhere from green to yellow, orange, or even red. The most important thing is that the color should be consistent all throughout and free of any strange discolouration or dark areas.

Skin Texture:

The surface of a fresh mango shouldn't have any blemishes, cuts, or bruises, and it should have a smooth texture all throughout. Mangoes that have a skin that is wrinkly or shriveled should be avoided since these characteristics may signal that the fruit has gone bad.

Weight:

A fresh mango should have a weight that is proportional to its size. This means that it is full of juicy, tasty meat and that it has a lot of it.

When Are Mangoes in Season?

Mangos are typically available in the United States from the month of May through the month of September. There is a possibility that imported mangoes will be accessible at other periods of the year.

Mango Flesh

The flesh of the mango is tender, juicy, and succulent, and it has a delectable texture that just about dissolves in your mouth. It is famous for its brilliant golden to orange-yellow hue, which, depending on the type of mango, can shift slightly from one shade to the next. Although the meat is fibrous, the fibers themselves are often smooth and soft, which makes it very simple to chew.

The flesh of a ripe mango has a taste that is reminiscent of tropical fruits and is sweet. Its sweetness and acidity are beautifully in tune with one another, resulting in a mouth feel that is just irresistible. The flavor profile might also have small differences based on the exact mango type; for example, certain varieties of mango include undertones of citrus or floral flavors, while other varieties have neither.

When compared to the flesh that is closer to the pit, the flesh that is closer to the skin tends to be slightly more solid and has a lower level of sweetness. It is not uncommon to discover a sizable, flat pit or seed in the center of the mango. This is the part of the fruit that has to be removed carefully before eating the mango.

The flesh of the mango is not only sweet but also chock full of many nutrients. In addition to providing dietary fiber and a number of other beneficial plant chemicals, it is also a rich source of vitamins, including vitamin C.

The flesh of the mango brings a blast of tropical taste and a touch of sunlight to any meal, whether it is consumed on its own, used in salads or salsas, blended into smoothies, or included in desserts. Mangoes may be found in Central and South America.

What to Look for in a Ripe Mango

To identify a ripe mango, pay attention to the following indicators:

- Color: The skin of a ripe mango can vary depending on the variety. However, a ripe mango will generally exhibit a vibrant hue, with a yellow or orange undertone. Some mangoes may also have a slight blush or pink spots.

- Firmness: Gently squeeze the mango to check for firmness. A ripe mango will yield slightly to gentle pressure, but it should not be overly soft.

- Aroma: A ripe mango will emit a sweet, fruity aroma from the stem end of the fruit. Sniff near the stem and make sure it has a pleasant scent.

What Color is a Ripe Mango?

The mature flesh of a mango can have a range of colors, depending on the type. Mangoes from the Tommy Atkins variety, for instance, get a dark red or purple hue when they are mature, but mangoes from the Kent variety acquire a golden color with a subtle blush.

Mangoes of the Alphonso kind are famous for their vivid yellow-orange color.

Familiarize yourself with the specific variety you're purchasing to determine its ideal color at peak ripeness.

How to Ripen an Unripe Mango

If you find yourself with an under ripe mango, you can use these simple steps to ripen it at home:

a. Place the mango in a brown paper bag: Put the unripe mango in a brown paper bag along with a ripe banana or apple. These fruits release ethylene gas, which speeds up the ripening process.

b. Wait a couple of days: Close the bag and leave it at room temperature for a couple of days. The mango will absorb the ethylene gas and ripen gradually.

c. Check for ripeness: After a few days, give the mango a gentle squeeze. If it yields slightly and has a sweet aroma, it is ready to be enjoyed.

Quick Tips for Handling Mangoes

When handling mangoes, keep these tips in mind:

- Use a sharp knife and a cutting board to cut the mango. Be careful while cutting around the mango seed.

- If you prefer not to cut the mango, you can scoop out the flesh using a large spoon or use a grid pattern and push the fruit upward to create mango pieces.

- To store cut mangoes, place them in an airtight container or wrap them in plastic wrap to maintain freshness.

Acquiring the necessary expertise via practice is the only way to successfully select a ripe mango. It is possible to select the ideal mango for your consumption by paying close attention to the mango's color, firmness, and aroma while making your selection. If you come across a mango that isn't quite ripe yet, you can follow the simple ripening procedure that involves a brown paper bag, an overripe banana, or an overripe apple. You will only need a few days to complete this procedure in order to obtain a mango that is fully ripe.

Refreshing Mango Smoothies

Mango and Banana Smoothie

1. Tropical Bliss Smoothie:

Ingredients:

- 1 cup frozen mango chunks
- 1 ripe banana
- 1/2 cup pineapple chunks
- 1/2 cup coconut milk
- 1/2 cup orange juice

Preparation:

1. Combine all ingredients in a blender.
2. Blend until smooth.
3. Pour into a glass and enjoy!

2. Mango Banana Green Smoothie:

Ingredients:

- 1 cup frozen mango chunks

- 1 ripe banana

- 1 cup spinach leaves

- 1/2 cup Greek yogurt

- 1/2 cup water

Preparation:

1. Add all ingredients to a blender.

2. Blend until the mixture is smooth.

3. Pour into a glass and savor the goodness!

3. Berry Mango Banana Smoothie:

Ingredients:

- 1 cup frozen mango chunks

- 1 ripe banana

- 1/2 cup mixed berries (strawberries, blueberries, raspberries)

- 1/2 cup almond milk

- 1 tablespoon honey

Preparation:

1. Blend mango, banana, berries, almond milk, and honey in a blender.

2. Blend until smooth and creamy.

3. Pour into a glass and relish the fruity blend.

4. Mango Banana Protein Smoothie:

Ingredients:

- 1 cup frozen mango chunks

- 1 ripe banana

- 1/2 cup plain Greek yogurt

- 1 scoop vanilla protein powder

- 1/2 cup water

Preparation:

1. Combine all ingredients in a blender.

2. Blend until the mixture is creamy and well combined.

3. Pour into a glass and enjoy your protein-packed smoothie!

5. Citrus Mango Banana Smoothie:

Ingredients:

- 1 cup frozen mango chunks

- 1 ripe banana

- 1/2 cup orange juice

- 1/4 cup lime juice

- 1/2 cup coconut water

Preparation:

1. Blend mango, banana, orange juice, lime juice, and coconut water in a blender.

2. Blend until smooth and refreshing.

3. Pour into a glass and sip away!

6. Mango Banana Oatmeal Smoothie:

Ingredients:

- 1 cup frozen mango chunks

- 1 ripe banana

- 1/2 cup rolled oats

- 1/2 cup milk (dairy or plant-based)

- 1 tablespoon chia seeds

Preparation:

1. Combine mango, banana, oats, milk, and chia seeds in a blender.

2. Blend until the oats are fully incorporated.

3. Pour into a glass, let it sit for a minute to thicken, and enjoy the hearty smoothie.

7. Minty Mango Banana Smoothie:

Ingredients:

- 1 cup frozen mango chunks
- 1 ripe banana
- 1/2 cup fresh mint leaves
- 1/2 cup coconut water
- 1 tablespoon lime juice

Preparation:

1. Blend mango, banana, mint leaves, coconut water, and lime juice in a blender.

2. Blend until smooth and minty fresh.

3. Pour into a glass and savor the coolness!

8. Mango Banana Avocado Smoothie:

Ingredients:

- 1 cup frozen mango chunks

- 1 ripe banana

- 1/2 avocado, peeled and pitted

- 1/2 cup almond milk

- 1 tablespoon honey

Preparation:

1. Combine mango, banana, avocado, almond milk, and honey in a blender.

2. Blend until creamy and luscious.

3. Pour into a glass and indulge in the rich flavors.

9. Spicy Mango Banana Smoothie:

Ingredients:

- 1 cup frozen mango chunks

- 1 ripe banana

- 1/2 cup orange juice

- 1/4 teaspoon cayenne pepper

- 1/2 cup water

Preparation:

1. Blend mango, banana, orange juice, cayenne pepper, and water in a blender.

2. Blend until smooth with a hint of spice.

3. Pour into a glass and enjoy the unique flavor kick!

10. Chocolate Mango Banana Smoothie:

Ingredients:

- 1 cup frozen mango chunks

- 1 ripe banana

- 2 tablespoons cocoa powder

- 1/2 cup chocolate almond milk

- 1/2 cup ice cubes

Preparation:

1. Combine mango, banana, cocoa powder, chocolate almond milk, and ice cubes in a blender.

2. Blend until smooth and chocolaty.

3. Pour into a glass and treat yourself to a delightful chocolate-infused smoothie!

Tropical Mango-Pineapple Smoothie

1. Classic Tropical Delight

Ingredients:

- 1 cup frozen mango chunks
- 1/2 cup frozen pineapple chunks
- 1 banana
- 1/2 cup Greek yogurt
- 1 cup coconut water
- Ice cubes (optional)

Preparation:

1. Combine all ingredients in a blender.
2. Blend until smooth.
3. Pour into a glass and enjoy!

2. Mango-Pineapple Paradise

Ingredients:

- 1 cup frozen mango chunks
- 1/2 cup frozen pineapple chunks
- 1/2 cup orange juice

- 1/2 cup coconut milk

- 1 tablespoon honey

- Ice cubes (optional)

Preparation:

1. Blend all the ingredients until creamy.

2. Taste and adjust sweetness if needed.

3. Pour into a glass and serve.

3. Protein-Packed Mango-Pineapple Smoothie

Ingredients:

- 1 cup frozen mango chunks

- 1/2 cup frozen pineapple chunks

- 1/2 cup vanilla protein powder

- 1 cup almond milk

- 1 tablespoon chia seeds

- Ice cubes (optional)

Preparation:

1. Combine all ingredients in a blender.

2. Blend until the mixture is smooth.

3. Pour into a glass and sprinkle some chia seeds on top.

4. Green Mango-Pineapple Bliss

Ingredients:

- 1 cup frozen mango chunks
- 1/2 cup frozen pineapple chunks
- Handful of spinach leaves
- 1/2 cup coconut water
- 1 tablespoon flaxseeds
- Ice cubes (optional)

Preparation:

1. Blend all the ingredients until the mixture is smooth and green.
2. Pour into a glass and enjoy a nutritious green smoothie.

5. Mango-Pineapple Citrus Splash

Ingredients:

- 1 cup frozen mango chunks
- 1/2 cup frozen pineapple chunks
- 1/2 cup orange juice

- 1/4 cup lime juice

- 1 tablespoon agave syrup

- Ice cubes (optional)

Preparation:

1. Blend all the ingredients until smooth.

2. Adjust sweetness with agave syrup if needed.

3. Pour into a glass and garnish with a slice of lime.

6. Coconut Mango-Pineapple Dream

Ingredients:

- 1 cup frozen mango chunks

- 1/2 cup frozen pineapple chunks

- 1/2 cup coconut milk

- 1/4 cup shredded coconut

- 1 tablespoon honey

- Ice cubes (optional)

Preparation:

1. Combine all ingredients in a blender.

2. Blend until creamy and smooth.

3. Pour into a glass and sprinkle shredded coconut on top.

7. Tropical Berry-Mango Fusion

Ingredients:

- 1 cup frozen mango chunks
- 1/2 cup frozen pineapple chunks
- 1/2 cup mixed berries (strawberries, blueberries, raspberries)
- 1/2 cup orange juice
- Ice cubes (optional)

Preparation:

1. Blend all ingredients until smooth.

2. Pour into a glass and enjoy the burst of tropical and berry flavors.

8. Minty Mango-Pineapple Cooler

Ingredients:

- 1 cup frozen mango chunks
- 1/2 cup frozen pineapple chunks
- Handful of fresh mint leaves

- 1 cup coconut water

- 1 tablespoon honey

- Ice cubes (optional)

Preparation:

1. Blend all ingredients until smooth.

2. Taste and adjust sweetness if needed.

3. Pour into a glass and garnish with a sprig of fresh mint.

9. Mango-Pineapple Protein Punch

Ingredients:

- 1 cup frozen mango chunks

- 1/2 cup frozen pineapple chunks

- 1/2 cup plain Greek yogurt

- 1 scoop vanilla protein powder

- 1 cup almond milk

- Ice cubes (optional)

Preparation:

1. Combine all ingredients in a blender.

2. Blend until the mixture is smooth and creamy.

3. Pour into a glass and enjoy the protein boost.

10. Spicy Mango-Pineapple Kick

Ingredients:

- 1 cup frozen mango chunks
- 1/2 cup frozen pineapple chunks
- 1/2 teaspoon cayenne pepper
- 1 tablespoon lime juice
- 1 cup coconut water
- Ice cubes (optional)

Preparation:

1. Blend all ingredients until smooth.

2. Adjust spiciness with cayenne pepper to taste.

3. Pour into a glass and enjoy the tropical-spicy fusion.

Mango Lassi

1. Classic Mango Lassi:

Ingredients:

- 1 cup ripe mango chunks
- 1 cup yogurt
- 1/2 cup milk
- 2 tablespoons honey
- Ice cubes (optional)

Preparation:

1. Combine mango chunks, yogurt, milk, and honey in a blender.
2. Blend until smooth.
3. Add ice cubes if desired and blend again.
4. Pour into a glass and serve chilled.

2. Tropical Mango Lassi:

Ingredients:

- 1 cup ripe mango chunks

- 1/2 cup pineapple chunks

- 1 cup coconut milk

- 1 tablespoon agave syrup

- Ice cubes (optional)

Preparation:

1. Blend mango chunks, pineapple chunks, coconut milk, and agave syrup until smooth.

2. Add ice cubes if desired and blend again.

3. Pour into a glass and enjoy the tropical flavors.

3. Berry Mango Lassi:

Ingredients:

- 1 cup ripe mango chunks

- 1/2 cup mixed berries (strawberries, blueberries, raspberries)

- 1 cup yogurt

- 1 tablespoon maple syrup

- Ice cubes (optional)

Preparation:

1. Blend mango chunks, mixed berries, yogurt, and maple syrup until well combined.

2. Add ice cubes if desired and blend again.

3. Pour into a glass and savor the fruity goodness.

4. Minty Mango Lassi:

Ingredients:

- 1 cup ripe mango chunks

- 1 cup yogurt

- 1/2 cup milk

- 1 tablespoon fresh mint leaves

- 2 tablespoons honey

- Ice cubes (optional)

Preparation:

1. Blend mango chunks, yogurt, milk, mint leaves, and honey until smooth.

2. Add ice cubes if desired and blend again.

3. Pour into a glass and enjoy the refreshing taste of mint.

5. Spiced Mango Lassi:

Ingredients:

- 1 cup ripe mango chunks
- 1 cup yogurt
- 1/2 cup milk
- 1/2 teaspoon ground cardamom
- 1/4 teaspoon ground cinnamon
- 2 tablespoons sugar
- Ice cubes (optional)

Preparation:

1. Blend mango chunks, yogurt, milk, cardamom, cinnamon, and sugar until well mixed.

2. Add ice cubes if desired and blend again.

3. Pour into a glass and savor the exotic spice blend.

6. Protein-Packed Mango Lassi:

Ingredients:

- 1 cup ripe mango chunks
- 1 cup Greek yogurt
- 1/2 cup almond milk
- 1 scoop vanilla protein powder
- 1 tablespoon honey
- Ice cubes (optional)

Preparation:

1. Blend mango chunks, Greek yogurt, almond milk, protein powder, and honey until smooth.

2. Add ice cubes if desired and blend again.

3. Pour into a glass for a nutritious and filling smoothie.

7. Avocado Mango Lassi:

Ingredients:

- 1 cup ripe mango chunks
- 1/2 ripe avocado, peeled and pitted
- 1 cup yogurt

- 1/2 cup milk

- 1 tablespoon agave syrup

- Ice cubes (optional)

Preparation:

1. Blend mango chunks, avocado, yogurt, milk, and agave syrup until creamy.

2. Add ice cubes if desired and blend again.

3. Pour into a glass for a unique and creamy twist.

8. Ginger Turmeric Mango Lassi:

Ingredients:

- 1 cup ripe mango chunks

- 1 cup yogurt

- 1/2 cup milk

- 1 teaspoon grated ginger

- 1/2 teaspoon ground turmeric

- 2 tablespoons honey

- Ice cubes (optional)

Preparation:

1. Blend mango chunks, yogurt, milk, ginger, turmeric, and honey until well combined.

2. Add ice cubes if desired and blend again.

3. Pour into a glass and enjoy the anti-inflammatory benefits of ginger and turmeric.

9. Coconut Mango Lassi:

Ingredients:

- 1 cup ripe mango chunks

- 1 cup coconut yogurt

- 1/2 cup coconut milk

- 1 tablespoon coconut flakes

- 1 tablespoon agave syrup

- Ice cubes (optional)

Preparation:

1. Blend mango chunks, coconut yogurt, coconut milk, coconut flakes, and agave syrup until smooth.

2. Add ice cubes if desired and blend again.

3. Pour into a glass for a tropical and coconut-infused treat.

10. Green Mango Lassi:

Ingredients:

- 1 cup ripe mango chunks
- 1 cup spinach leaves
- 1 cup yogurt
- 1/2 cup milk
- 1 tablespoon honey
- Ice cubes (optional)

Preparation:

1. Blend mango chunks, spinach leaves, yogurt, milk, and honey until the mixture turns green and smooth.

2. Add ice cubes if desired and blend again.

3. Pour into a glass for a nutrient-packed green smoothie with a hint of mango sweetness.

Savory Mango Salads

Mango Avocado Salad

Ingredients

6 Servings

⅓ Cup extra-virgin olive oil

⅓ Cup fresh blood orange juice

¼ cup fresh lime juice

1 Tbsp. honey

1 Tbsp. Diamond Crystal or 1¾ tsp. Morton kosher salt

½ tsp. freshly ground black pepper

1 shallot, finely chopped

2 Tbsp. finely chopped cilantro

4 blood oranges, peel and white pith removed, flesh sliced into irregular pieces

2 mangoes, peeled, sliced

2 avocados, peeled, sliced

1 cup halved cherry tomatoes

Preparation

1. **Step 1**

Whisk oil, blood orange juice, lime juice, honey, salt, and pepper in a small bowl to combine; mix in shallot and cilantro.

Step 2

Arrange blood oranges, mangoes, avocados, and cherry tomatoes on a platter. Drizzle dressing over.

Spicy Mango and Black Bean Salad

Spicy Mango and Black Bean Salad is a delightful and refreshing dish that combines the sweetness of ripe mangoes with the earthiness of black beans, all kicked up with a bit of spice. Here's a simple recipe for you to try:

Ingredients:

- 1 can (15 ounces) black beans, drained and rinsed

- 2 ripe mangoes, peeled, pitted, and diced

- 1 red bell pepper, diced

- 1/2 red onion, finely chopped

- 1/4 cup fresh cilantro, chopped

- Juice of 2 limes

- 2 tablespoons olive oil

- 1 teaspoon honey or agave nectar (optional, for added sweetness)

- 1 teaspoon ground cumin

- 1/2 teaspoon chili powder (adjust to taste for spiciness)

- Salt and black pepper to taste

- Optional toppings: avocado slices, sliced jalapeños

Instructions:

1. **Prepare Ingredients:** Rinse and drain the black beans. Peel, pit, and dice the ripe mangoes. Dice the red bell pepper,

finely chop the red onion, and chop the fresh cilantro.

2. **Make Dressing:** In a small bowl, whisk together lime juice, olive oil, honey or agave nectar (if using), ground cumin, chili powder, salt, and black pepper. Adjust the seasonings to taste.

3. **Combine Ingredients:** In a large mixing bowl, combine the black beans, diced mangoes, red bell pepper, red onion, and cilantro.

4. **Toss with Dressing:** Pour the dressing over the salad ingredients and gently toss until everything is well coated.

5. **Chill:** Cover the bowl and refrigerate for at least 30 minutes to allow the flavors to meld.

6. **Serve:** Just before serving, give the salad a final toss. Optionally, top with avocado slices and sliced jalapeños for extra flavor and texture.

7. **Enjoy:** Serve the spicy mango and black bean salad as a refreshing side

dish, or enjoy it on its own. It's perfect for picnics, barbecues, or as a light and healthy lunch.

Grilled Chicken and Mango Salad

Ingredients:

For the Grilled Chicken:

- 2 boneless, skinless chicken breasts
- 2 tablespoons olive oil
- 1 teaspoon garlic powder
- 1 teaspoon paprika
- Salt and pepper to taste

For the Salad:

- 2 ripe mangoes, peeled, pitted, and diced
- 1 cucumber, diced
- 1 red bell pepper, diced
- 1/4 red onion, thinly sliced

- 1/4 cup fresh cilantro, chopped

For the Dressing:

- 3 tablespoons olive oil

- 2 tablespoons lime juice

- 1 tablespoon honey

- Salt and pepper to taste

Instructions:

1. **Marinate the Chicken:**

   - In a bowl, mix olive oil, garlic powder, paprika, salt, and pepper.

   - Coat the chicken breasts with the marinade and let them marinate for at least 30 minutes in the refrigerator.

2. **Grill the Chicken:**

   - Preheat the grill to medium-high heat.

   - Grill the chicken breasts for about 6-8 minutes per side or

until they reach an internal
temperature of 165°F (74°C).

- Once cooked, let the chicken
  rest for a few minutes before
  slicing it into strips.

3. **Prepare the Salad:**

- In a large bowl, combine diced
  mangoes, cucumber, red bell
  pepper, red onion, and cilantro.

4. **Make the Dressing:**

- In a small bowl, whisk together
  olive oil, lime juice, honey, salt,
  and pepper until well combined.

5. **Assemble the Salad:**

- Add the grilled chicken strips to
  the salad.

- Drizzle the dressing over the
  salad and toss gently to combine,
  ensuring the salad is evenly
  coated with the dressing.

6. **Serve:**

- Divide the salad among plates and serve immediately.

Delicious Mango Salsas

Classic Mango Salsa

Classic Mango Salsa is a delicious and refreshing condiment that pairs well with various dishes, especially grilled meats, seafood, or as a dip with tortilla chips. Here's a simple recipe for you to make classic mango salsa at home:

Ingredients:

- 2 ripe mangoes, diced
- 1/2 red onion, finely chopped
- 1 red bell pepper, diced
- 1 jalapeño pepper, finely chopped (seeds and ribs removed for less heat, if desired)
- 1/4 cup fresh cilantro, chopped
- Juice of 2 limes
- Salt and pepper to taste

Instructions:

1. **Prepare the Ingredients:** Peel and
   dice the ripe mangoes. Finely chop the
   red onion, red bell pepper, jalapeño
   pepper, and cilantro.

2. **Combine Ingredients:** In a mixing
   bowl, combine the diced mangoes,
   chopped red onion, diced red bell
   pepper, chopped jalapeño pepper, and
   chopped cilantro.

3. **Add Lime Juice:** Squeeze the juice of
   two limes over the mixture. Adjust the
   amount of lime juice to your taste
   preferences.

4. **Season:** Season the salsa with salt and
   pepper to taste. Be mindful of the salt,
   as the chips you might be serving with
   the salsa are often salted.

5. **Mix Well:** Gently toss all the
   ingredients together until well
   combined. Make sure the lime juice and
   seasonings are evenly distributed.

6. **Chill (Optional):** For enhanced
   flavors, you can refrigerate the salsa for
   at least 30 minutes before serving. This

also allows the ingredients to meld together.

7. **Serve:** Serve the classic mango salsa with grilled chicken, fish, tacos, or as a refreshing dip with tortilla chips.

Mango and Tomato Salsa

Mango and tomato salsa is a delicious and refreshing condiment that combines the sweetness of ripe mangoes with the tanginess of tomatoes. It's a versatile accompaniment that pairs well with grilled meats, fish, tacos, or as a topping for salads. Here's a simple recipe for making mango and tomato salsa:

Ingredients:

- 1 large ripe mango, peeled, pitted, and diced

- 1 cup cherry tomatoes, halved (you can also use regular tomatoes, diced)

- 1/2 red onion, finely chopped

- 1 jalapeño pepper, seeded and finely chopped (adjust to taste)

- 1/4 cup fresh cilantro, chopped

- Juice of 1 lime

- Salt and pepper to taste

Instructions:

1. **Prepare the Ingredients:** Peel and dice the ripe mango. Halve the cherry tomatoes (or dice regular tomatoes), finely chop the red onion, jalapeño pepper, and fresh cilantro.

2. **Combine Ingredients:** In a bowl, combine the diced mango, halved cherry tomatoes, chopped red onion, jalapeño pepper, and cilantro.

3. **Add Lime Juice:** Squeeze the juice of one lime over the mixture. Lime juice adds a citrusy brightness to the salsa.

4. **Season with Salt and Pepper:** Season the salsa with salt and pepper to taste. Start with a small amount and adjust according to your preference.

5. **Mix Well:** Gently toss all the ingredients together until well

combined. Be careful not to mash the mango; you want to keep some texture.

6. **Chill (Optional):** If time allows, cover the salsa and let it chill in the refrigerator for about 30 minutes. Chilling enhances the flavors.

7. **Serve:** Once chilled (if desired), give the salsa a final stir and serve. It's great on its own as a dip with tortilla chips, or as a topping for grilled chicken, fish, tacos, or salads.

Shrimp and Mango Salsa

Shrimp and mango salsa is a delicious and refreshing dish that combines the flavors of succulent shrimp with the sweetness of ripe mango and the freshness of various herbs and vegetables. Here's a simple recipe for you to try:

Ingredients:

For the Shrimp:

- 1 pound large shrimp, peeled and deveined

- 1 tablespoon olive oil

- 1 teaspoon smoked paprika

- Salt and black pepper to taste

- Lime wedges for serving

For the Mango Salsa:

- 2 ripe mangoes, peeled, pitted, and diced

- 1/2 red onion, finely chopped

- 1 red bell pepper, diced

- 1 jalapeño pepper, seeded and finely chopped (adjust to taste)

- 1/4 cup fresh cilantro, chopped

- Juice of 2 limes

- Salt and black pepper to taste

Instructions:

1. Prepare the Shrimp:

   1. In a bowl, combine the shrimp with olive oil, smoked paprika, salt, and

black pepper. Toss until the shrimp are
evenly coated.

2. Heat a large skillet over medium-high
   heat. Add the shrimp and cook for 2-3
   minutes per side or until they turn pink
   and opaque.

3. Remove the shrimp from the skillet
   and set aside.

2. Make the Mango Salsa:

1. In a large bowl, combine diced
   mangoes, red onion, red bell pepper,
   jalapeño, and cilantro.

2. Add lime juice and gently toss the
   ingredients together.

3. Season with salt and black pepper to
   taste.

3. Assemble the Dish:

1. Serve the cooked shrimp on a platter or
   individual plates.

2. Spoon the mango salsa over the
   shrimp.

3. Garnish with additional cilantro and
   lime wedges.

4. Serve immediately and enjoy!

Sweet and Spicy Mango Chutneys

Traditional Mango Chutney

Ingredients:

- 2 large ripe mangoes, peeled, pitted, and diced
- 1 cup granulated sugar
- 1/2 cup white vinegar
- 1 small onion, finely chopped
- 1/4 cup raisins
- 1/4 teaspoon ground ginger
- 1/4 teaspoon ground cinnamon
- 1/4 teaspoon ground cloves
- 1/4 teaspoon chili powder (adjust to taste for spice)
- Salt to taste

Instructions:

1. **Prepare the Mangoes:** Peel, pit, and dice the ripe mangoes. Ensure they are ripe but still firm.

2. **Cook the Ingredients:** In a saucepan, combine the diced mangoes, sugar, vinegar, chopped onion, raisins, ground ginger, ground cinnamon, ground cloves, chili powder, and a pinch of salt.

3. **Simmer:** Bring the mixture to a boil over medium heat, stirring occasionally to dissolve the sugar. Once it boils, reduce the heat to low and let it simmer.

4. **Cook Until Thickened:** Allow the chutney to simmer for about 45 minutes to 1 hour, or until it has thickened to your desired consistency. Stir occasionally to prevent sticking.

5. **Adjust Seasoning:** Taste the chutney and adjust the seasoning as needed. You can add more sugar if you prefer it sweeter or more chili powder for extra spice.

6. **Cool and Store:** Once the chutney has thickened and reached the desired flavor, remove it from the heat and let it cool. It will continue to thicken as it cools. Once cooled, transfer it to sterilized jars and store in the refrigerator.

7. **Serve:** Traditional mango chutney is ready to be served. It's a versatile condiment that adds a burst of flavor to various dishes.

Mango Ginger Chutney

Ingredients:

- 1 cup mango ginger, peeled and finely chopped

- 1 cup raw mango, peeled and finely chopped

- 1 cup jaggery (or sugar)

- 1 tablespoon oil

- 1 teaspoon mustard seeds

- 1/2 teaspoon fenugreek seeds

- 1/2 teaspoon cumin seeds

- 1/4 teaspoon asafoetida (hing)

- 1-2 dried red chillies, broken into pieces

- 1/2 teaspoon turmeric powder

- Salt to taste

- Water, as needed

Instructions:

1. **Prepare the Ingredients:** Peel and finely chop the mango ginger and raw mango. If you're using jaggery, grate it to make it easier to dissolve in the chutney.

2. **Cooking the Chutney:**

   - Heat oil in a pan over medium heat.

   - Add mustard seeds, fenugreek seeds, cumin seeds, asafoetida, and dried red chillies. Sauté until the mustard seeds start to splutter.

- Add the chopped mango ginger and raw mango to the pan. Cook for a few minutes until they start to soften.

3. **Add Spices:**

   - Add turmeric powder and salt to the mixture. Stir well to combine the spices evenly.

4. **Sweetening the Chutney:**

   - Add the jaggery (or sugar) to the pan. Mix well and let it melt, creating a sweet and tangy base for the chutney.

5. **Simmer:**

   - Reduce the heat to low and let the chutney simmer. Stir occasionally and cook until the mixture thickens to your desired consistency.

6. **Adjust Consistency:**

   - If the chutney is too thick, you can add a little water to achieve the desired consistency.

Remember that it will thicken slightly as it cools.

7. **Cool and Store:**

   - Allow the chutney to cool completely before transferring it to a clean, dry jar. It can be stored in the refrigerator for a few weeks.

Spiced Mango and Pineapple Chutney

Spiced Mango and Pineapple Chutney is a delightful and flavorful condiment that adds a sweet and tangy kick to a variety of dishes. It's a versatile accompaniment that pairs well with grilled meats, curries, sandwiches, and more. Here's a simple recipe for you to try:

Ingredients:

- 2 cups diced mango (ripe)

- 1 cup diced pineapple

- 1/2 cup finely chopped red onion

- 1/4 cup raisins
- 1/4 cup chopped dates
- 1/2 cup brown sugar
- 1/2 cup apple cider vinegar
- 1 teaspoon grated ginger
- 1 teaspoon minced garlic
- 1/2 teaspoon mustard seeds
- 1/2 teaspoon cumin seeds
- 1/4 teaspoon turmeric powder
- 1/4 teaspoon red chili flakes (adjust to taste)
- Salt to taste

Instructions:

1. **Prepare the Fruits:**
   - Peel and dice the mango.
   - Dice the pineapple.
   - Finely chop the red onion.

2. **Cooking the Chutney:**

- In a large saucepan, combine the diced mango, pineapple, red onion, raisins, dates, brown sugar, apple cider vinegar, grated ginger, and minced garlic.

3. **Tempering:**

   - In a small pan, heat a bit of oil over medium heat.

   - Add mustard seeds and cumin seeds. Allow them to splutter.

   - Add turmeric powder and red chili flakes. Stir for a few seconds.

4. **Combine:**

   - Pour the tempering mixture into the large saucepan with the fruit mixture.

5. **Cooking:**

   - Place the saucepan over medium heat and bring the mixture to a boil.

   - Reduce the heat and simmer for about 30-40 minutes, stirring occasionally, until the chutney thickens and the fruits are soft.

6. **Adjust Seasoning:**

   - Taste the chutney and adjust the salt and sweetness according to your preference.

7. **Cooling and Storage:**

   - Allow the chutney to cool to room temperature before transferring it to sterilized jars.

   - Store in the refrigerator. The flavors will continue to develop over time.

8. **Serving:**

   - Serve the spiced mango and pineapple chutney as a condiment with grilled meats, curries, sandwiches, or cheese.

Mango Desserts for Every Occasion

Mango Coconut Rice Pudding

Ingredients:

- 1 cup Arborio rice
- 1 can (13.5 oz) coconut milk
- 2 cups whole milk
- 1/2 cup sugar (adjust to taste)
- 1 teaspoon vanilla extract
- 1/4 teaspoon salt
- 1 ripe mango, peeled and diced
- Shredded coconut for garnish (optional)

Instructions:

1. **Rinse the Rice:**
   - Rinse the Arborio rice under cold water until the water runs

clear. This helps remove excess starch.

2. **Cook the Rice:**

   - In a medium-sized saucepan, combine the rinsed rice, coconut milk, whole milk, sugar, vanilla extract, and salt.

   - Bring the mixture to a simmer over medium heat, stirring frequently.

3. **Simmer:**

   - Reduce the heat to low and let the rice mixture simmer gently. Stir occasionally to prevent the rice from sticking to the bottom of the pan.

4. **Cook Until Thickened:**

   - Continue cooking until the rice absorbs most of the liquid, and the mixture thickens to a creamy consistency. This may take about 20-25 minutes.

5. **Add Mango:**

- Once the rice pudding reaches the desired consistency, remove it from the heat. Allow it to cool slightly.

- Gently fold in the diced mango.

6. **Chill:**

   - Transfer the rice pudding to a serving dish or individual serving bowls. Cover and refrigerate until chilled.

7. **Serve:**

   - Before serving, you can garnish the mango coconut rice pudding with additional diced mango and shredded coconut if desired.

8. **Enjoy:**

   - Serve the mango coconut rice pudding cold and enjoy the tropical flavors!

Mango Cheesecake Bars

Mango cheesecake bars are a delightful and tropical twist on the classic cheesecake. Here's a simple recipe for you to try:

Ingredients:

For the Crust:

- 1 1/2 cups graham cracker crumbs
- 1/3 cup melted butter
- 1/4 cup granulated sugar

For the Cheesecake Filling:

- 3 packages (24 ounces) cream cheese, softened
- 1 cup granulated sugar
- 3 large eggs
- 1 teaspoon vanilla extract
- 1 cup mango puree (fresh or canned)
- 1/4 cup all-purpose flour

For the Mango Swirl:

- 1/2 cup mango puree

- 2 tablespoons granulated sugar

Instructions:

1. Preheat the Oven:

Preheat your oven to 325°F (163°C). Line a 9x13-inch baking dish with parchment paper, leaving an overhang on the sides for easy removal.

2. Prepare the Crust:

In a bowl, combine the graham cracker crumbs, melted butter, and 1/4 cup of sugar. Press the mixture into the bottom of the prepared baking dish to form an even crust. Bake for about 10 minutes or until the crust is set.

3. Make the Cheesecake Filling:

a. In a large mixing bowl, beat the cream cheese until smooth. b. Add the sugar and beat until well combined. c. Add the eggs one at a time, beating well after each addition. d. Mix in the vanilla extract. e. Add the mango puree and flour, and beat until smooth and well combined.

4. Pour and Swirl:

Pour the cheesecake filling over the crust in the baking dish.

In a small bowl, mix together 1/2 cup of mango puree and 2 tablespoons of sugar. Spoon dollops of the mango swirl mixture over the cheesecake filling. Use a knife or toothpick to swirl the mango mixture into the cheesecake batter, creating a marbled effect.

5. Bake:

Bake in the preheated oven for 40-45 minutes or until the center is set. The edges should be slightly golden.

6. Cool and Chill:

Allow the mango cheesecake bars to cool completely in the baking dish on a wire rack. Once cooled, refrigerate for at least 4 hours or overnight.

7. Slice and Serve:

Lift the chilled cheesecake out of the baking dish using the parchment paper overhang. Cut into bars, and serve chilled. Optionally, you can garnish with fresh mango slices or a sprinkle of powdered sugar before serving.

No-Bake Mango Pie

No-bake mango pie is a delicious and easy-to-make dessert that celebrates the sweet and tropical flavor of mangoes. Here's a simple recipe for a no-bake mango pie:

Ingredients:

For the Crust:

- 1 1/2 cups graham cracker crumbs
- 1/3 cup melted butter
- 1/4 cup sugar

For the Filling:

- 3 large ripe mangoes, peeled, pitted, and diced
- 1/2 cup sugar (adjust according to sweetness of mangoes)
- 1 tablespoon lemon juice
- 1 teaspoon gelatin powder (dissolved in 2 tablespoons of hot water)
- 1 cup whipped cream

For Garnish (optional):

- Sliced mangoes

- Mint leaves

Instructions:

1. Prepare the Crust:

a. In a bowl, combine the graham cracker crumbs, melted butter, and sugar. b. Press the mixture into the bottom of a pie pan to form the crust. You can use the back of a spoon to make it smooth and compact. c. Place the crust in the refrigerator to set while you prepare the filling.

2. Make the Filling:

a. In a blender or food processor, puree the diced mangoes until smooth. b. Add sugar and lemon juice to the mango puree and blend again until well combined. c. In a small bowl, dissolve the gelatin powder in hot water. Allow it to cool slightly. d. Add the dissolved gelatin to the mango mixture and blend again. e. In a separate bowl, whip the cream until stiff peaks form. f. Gently fold the whipped cream into the mango mixture until well combined.

3. Assemble the Pie:

a. Take the prepared crust out of the refrigerator. b. Pour the mango filling into the crust, spreading it evenly. c. Smooth the top with a spatula. d. Place the pie back in the refrigerator and let it set for at least 4 hours or until firm.

4. Garnish (Optional):

a. Before serving, garnish the pie with sliced mangoes and mint leaves for a fresh and decorative touch.

5. Serve and Enjoy:

a. Once the pie is set, slice and serve chilled. Enjoy the tropical goodness of your no-bake mango pie!

Mango-infused Main Courses

Mango Chicken Curry

Mango chicken curry is a delicious and flavorful dish that combines the sweetness of ripe mangoes with the savory and spicy flavors of a curry. Here's a simple recipe for you to try:

Ingredients:

- 1.5 lbs (about 700g) boneless, skinless chicken thighs, cut into bite-sized pieces

- 2 ripe mangoes, peeled, pitted, and diced

- 1 large onion, finely chopped

- 3 cloves garlic, minced

- 1 tablespoon ginger, grated

- 1 can (14 oz/400ml) coconut milk

- 1 can (14 oz/400g) diced tomatoes

- 2 tablespoons curry powder

- 1 teaspoon turmeric

- 1 teaspoon cumin

- 1 teaspoon coriander

- 1/2 teaspoon chili powder (adjust to taste)

- Salt and pepper to taste

- 2 tablespoons cooking oil

- Fresh cilantro, chopped (for garnish)

- Cooked rice (for serving)

Instructions:

1. **Marinate the chicken:** In a bowl, combine the chicken pieces with curry powder, turmeric, cumin, coriander, chili powder, salt, and pepper. Mix well and let it marinate for at least 30 minutes.

2. **Sauté the aromatics:** Heat the cooking oil in a large skillet or pan over medium heat. Add chopped onions and sauté until they become translucent.

Add minced garlic and grated ginger, sauté for another minute until fragrant.

3. **Cook the chicken:** Add the marinated chicken to the pan and cook until the chicken is browned on all sides.

4. **Add tomatoes and coconut milk:** Pour in the diced tomatoes and coconut milk. Stir well to combine. Bring the mixture to a simmer and let it cook for about 15-20 minutes, or until the chicken is cooked through.

5. **Add mangoes:** Gently stir in the diced mangoes and cook for an additional 5-10 minutes, allowing the flavors to meld together. Adjust the seasoning if necessary.

6. **Serve:** Once the chicken is cooked and the sauce has thickened, remove the curry from heat. Serve the mango chicken curry over cooked rice and garnish with chopped fresh cilantro.

Grilled Mango Glazed Salmon

Grilled Mango Glazed Salmon is a delightful dish that combines the richness of salmon with the sweetness of mango glaze. Here's a simple recipe for you to try:

Ingredients:

- 4 salmon fillets
- 1 ripe mango, peeled and diced
- 2 tablespoons soy sauce
- 2 tablespoons honey
- 1 tablespoon Dijon mustard
- 1 tablespoon olive oil
- 2 cloves garlic, minced
- 1 teaspoon grated ginger
- Salt and pepper to taste
- Fresh cilantro or parsley for garnish (optional)

Instructions:

1. **Prepare the Mango Glaze:**

- In a blender or food processor, combine the diced mango, soy sauce, honey, Dijon mustard, olive oil, minced garlic, and grated ginger. Blend until smooth.

2. **Marinate the Salmon:**

   - Place the salmon fillets in a shallow dish or a resealable plastic bag.

   - Pour half of the mango glaze over the salmon, making sure to coat each fillet evenly. Reserve the other half of the glaze for later use.

   - Marinate the salmon for at least 30 minutes in the refrigerator, allowing the flavors to infuse.

3. **Preheat the Grill:**

   - Preheat your grill to medium-high heat. Make sure to clean and oil the grates to prevent sticking.

4. **Grill the Salmon:**

- Remove the salmon from the marinade and discard the used marinade.

- Place the salmon fillets on the preheated grill, skin side down. Grill for about 4-5 minutes per side or until the salmon easily flakes with a fork. Baste the salmon with the reserved mango glaze during grilling.

5. **Serve:**

  - Once the salmon is cooked through, transfer it to a serving platter.

  - Drizzle the remaining mango glaze over the grilled salmon.

  - Garnish with fresh cilantro or parsley if desired.

6. **Optional: Sides:**

  - Serve the Grilled Mango Glazed Salmon with your favorite sides, such as rice, quinoa, or a fresh salad.

Vegetarian Mango Stir-Fry

Certainly! Here's a simple recipe for Vegetarian Mango Stir-Fry:

Ingredients:

- 1 large ripe mango, peeled, pitted, and sliced

- 1 cup broccoli florets

- 1 red bell pepper, sliced

- 1 yellow bell pepper, sliced

- 1 carrot, julienned

- 1 cup snap peas, trimmed

- 1/2 cup sliced red onion

- 2 cloves garlic, minced

- 1 tablespoon ginger, grated

- 1/4 cup soy sauce

- 2 tablespoons hoisin sauce

- 1 tablespoon rice vinegar

- 1 tablespoon sesame oil

- 2 tablespoons vegetable oil

- 1/4 cup chopped cilantro (for garnish)

- Cooked rice or noodles (for serving)

Instructions:

1. **Prepare the Vegetables:**

   - Slice the mango, bell peppers, and red onion.

   - Julienne the carrot.

   - Trim the snap peas.

   - Mince the garlic and grate the ginger.

2. **Make the Sauce:**

   - In a small bowl, mix together soy sauce, hoisin sauce, and rice vinegar. Set aside.

3. **Stir-Fry:**

   - Heat vegetable oil in a large wok or skillet over medium-high heat.

   - Add minced garlic and grated ginger. Sauté for about 30 seconds until fragrant.

- Add broccoli, bell peppers,
  carrot, snap peas, and red onion
  to the wok. Stir-fry for 3-5
  minutes until the vegetables are
  slightly tender but still crisp.

- Add the sliced mango to the
  wok and stir-fry for an additional
  2 minutes.

4. **Add the Sauce:**

- Pour the prepared sauce over the
  vegetables and mango. Stir well
  to coat everything evenly.

5. **Finish Cooking:**

- Drizzle sesame oil over the stir-
  fry and toss to combine.

- Cook for an additional 2-3
  minutes until everything is
  heated through, and the flavors
  meld together.

6. **Serve:**

- Serve the Vegetarian Mango Stir-
  Fry over cooked rice or noodles.

- Garnish with chopped cilantro.

Homemade Mango Ice Cream and Popsicles

Mango Sorbet

Mango sorbet is a delicious frozen dessert made primarily from ripe mangoes. It's a refreshing and fruity option, perfect for hot days or as a light and sweet treat after a meal. Here's a simple recipe for making mango sorbet at home:

Ingredients:

- 4 cups ripe mangoes, peeled, pitted, and chopped (about 4-5 mangoes)

- 1 cup granulated sugar (adjust to taste, depending on the sweetness of the mangoes)

- 1/4 cup fresh lime or lemon juice

- 1 cup water

Instructions:

1. **Prepare the Mango:**

    - Peel, pit, and chop the ripe
      mangoes.

2. **Make Simple Syrup:**

    - In a small saucepan, combine the
      sugar and water. Heat over
      medium heat, stirring until the
      sugar dissolves. This creates a
      simple syrup.

    - Remove from heat and let it
      cool.

3. **Blend the Ingredients:**

    - In a blender or food processor,
      combine the chopped mangoes
      and lime/lemon juice.

    - Blend until smooth.

    - Add the cooled simple syrup to
      the mango puree and blend
      again until well combined.

4. **Chill the Mixture:**

- Pour the mango mixture into a bowl and refrigerate for at least 2 hours or until thoroughly chilled.

5. **Freeze the Sorbet:**

   - Once the mixture is chilled, transfer it to an ice cream maker and churn according to the manufacturer's instructions.

   - If you don't have an ice cream maker, you can pour the mixture into a shallow dish and place it in the freezer. Stir the mixture every 30 minutes for the first 2-3 hours to prevent ice crystals from forming.

6. **Serve:**

   - Once the sorbet has reached a firm, scoopable consistency, transfer it to a lidded container and freeze until ready to serve.

7. **Garnish (optional):**

   - Garnish the mango sorbet with fresh mint leaves or a slice of lime for added freshness.

Creamy Mango Ice Cream

Creamy mango ice cream is a delightful and refreshing frozen dessert that captures the sweet and tropical flavor of ripe mangoes. Here's a simple recipe you can try at home:

Ingredients:

- 2 cups ripe mango, peeled, pitted, and chopped

- 1 cup granulated sugar

- 2 cups heavy cream

- 1 cup whole milk

- 1 teaspoon vanilla extract

- Pinch of salt

- Optional: 1 tablespoon fresh lime or lemon juice (to enhance the mango flavor)

Instructions:

1. **Prepare the Mango:** Peel and chop the ripe mangoes into small pieces.

2. **Puree the Mango:** Place the chopped mango in a blender or food processor and blend until you have a smooth puree. If desired, you can add fresh lime or lemon juice to enhance the mango flavor. Set aside.

3. **Prepare the Ice Cream Base:** In a mixing bowl, whisk together the granulated sugar, heavy cream, whole milk, vanilla extract, and a pinch of salt until the sugar is dissolved.

4. **Combine Mango Puree and Ice Cream Base:** Gently fold the mango puree into the ice cream base until well combined. Make sure the mixture is smooth and evenly mixed.

5. **Chill the Mixture:** Cover the bowl with plastic wrap and refrigerate for at least 4 hours or overnight. This allows the flavors to meld and the mixture to chill thoroughly.

6. **Churn the Ice Cream:** Once the mixture is well chilled, pour it into an ice cream maker and churn according to the manufacturer's instructions.

7. **Transfer and Freeze:** Transfer the churned ice cream to a lidded container and freeze for an additional 4 hours or until the ice cream reaches the desired consistency.

8. **Serve and Enjoy:** Scoop the creamy mango ice cream into bowls or cones and enjoy! You can garnish it with additional mango slices or a sprinkle of toasted coconut for added texture.

Mango Coconut Popsicles

Mango Coconut Popsicles are a delicious and refreshing treat, perfect for hot summer days. Here's a simple recipe for you to try:

Ingredients:

- 2 ripe mangoes, peeled and diced

- 1 cup coconut milk

- 1/4 cup honey or agave nectar (adjust to taste)

- 1 teaspoon vanilla extract

- 1/2 cup shredded coconut (optional, for added texture)

Instructions:

1. **Prepare the Mango:**

   - Peel and dice the ripe mangoes.

2. **Blend the Ingredients:**

   - In a blender, combine the diced mangoes, coconut milk, honey or agave nectar, and vanilla extract.

   - Blend until you have a smooth and creamy mixture.

3. **Add Shredded Coconut (Optional):**

   - If you want to add some texture to your popsicles, stir in the shredded coconut into the blended mixture. This step is optional and can be skipped if you prefer a smoother texture.

4. **Fill Popsicle Molds:**

   - Pour the mango-coconut mixture into popsicle molds.

Leave a little space at the top to allow for expansion as the popsicles freeze.

5. **Insert Sticks:**

   - Place the sticks into the molds. If your popsicle mold comes with a cover, put it on and insert the sticks through the designated holes.

6. **Freeze:**

   - Place the popsicle molds in the freezer and let them freeze for at least 4-6 hours, or until completely solid.

7. **Enjoy:**

   - Once the popsicles are fully frozen, remove them from the molds by running warm water over the outside of the mold to loosen the popsicles.

   - Enjoy your homemade Mango Coconut Popsicles!

Mango Beverages for All Ages

Mango Iced Tea

Mango iced tea is a refreshing and flavorful beverage that combines the sweetness of ripe mangoes with the briskness of black tea. Here's a simple recipe for making mango iced tea:

Ingredients:

1. Black tea bags (2 to 3, depending on your preferred strength)

2. Ripe mangoes (2 medium-sized, peeled and diced)

3. Water (4 cups for steeping tea, additional water for dilution)

4. Ice cubes

5. Sugar or sweetener (optional, to taste)

6. Mint leaves for garnish (optional)

7. Lemon slices for garnish (optional)

Instructions:

1. Boil 4 cups of water. Once the water is boiling, add the black tea bags and steep for about 3-5 minutes, or according to the instructions on the tea package. The longer you steep, the stronger the tea will be.

2. While the tea is steeping, puree the diced mangoes in a blender until smooth. You can adjust the amount of mango puree based on your taste preferences.

3. After steeping, remove the tea bags from the water and let the tea cool to room temperature. You can speed up the cooling process by placing the pot in the refrigerator.

4. Once the tea has cooled, combine it with the mango puree. Mix well to ensure the flavors are evenly distributed.

5. Taste the mixture and add sugar or sweetener if desired. Stir until the sweetener is fully dissolved.

6. Refrigerate the mango tea mixture for at least 1-2 hours to chill.

7. When ready to serve, fill glasses with ice cubes and pour the chilled mango tea over the ice.

8. Garnish with mint leaves and lemon slices if desired.

Sparkling Mango Lemonade

Sparkling Mango Lemonade is a refreshing and delightful beverage that combines the tropical sweetness of mango with the tartness of lemon, all topped off with the effervescence of sparkling water. Here's a simple recipe for you to try:

Ingredients:

- 1 cup fresh mango puree (you can use ripe mangoes and blend them)

- 1/2 cup fresh lemon juice (about 3-4 lemons)

- 1/2 cup simple syrup (adjust according to your sweetness preference)

- 2 cups sparkling water

- Ice cubes

- Lemon slices and mint leaves for garnish

Instructions:

1. **Prepare Simple Syrup:**

    - In a small saucepan, combine equal parts water and sugar.

    - Heat over medium heat, stirring until the sugar completely dissolves.

    - Allow it to cool, and you have your simple syrup.

2. **Prepare Mango Puree:**

    - Peel and dice ripe mangoes.

    - Place the mango pieces in a blender and blend until smooth.

- If the puree is too thick, you can add a little water to achieve the desired consistency.

3. **Mix Ingredients:**

   - In a large pitcher, combine the fresh mango puree, lemon juice, and simple syrup.

   - Stir the mixture well to ensure the flavors are evenly distributed.

4. **Add Sparkling Water:**

   - Just before serving, pour the sparkling water into the pitcher and gently stir to combine.

   - You can adjust the amount of sparkling water based on your preference for the level of fizziness.

5. **Serve:**

   - Fill glasses with ice cubes and pour the sparkling mango lemonade over the ice.

6. **Garnish:**

- Garnish each glass with a slice of lemon on the rim and a sprig of mint for a fresh aroma.

7. **Enjoy:**

   - Stir the drink gently before sipping to make sure all the flavors are well-mixed.

   - Enjoy your Sparkling Mango Lemonade on a hot day or whenever you crave a tropical and fizzy drink!

Mango Mojito

A Mango Mojito is a delicious and refreshing tropical twist on the classic Mojito cocktail. Here's a simple recipe for you to try:

Ingredients:

- 1 cup fresh mango chunks (about 1 large mango)

- 10 fresh mint leaves, plus extra for garnish

- 1 tablespoon sugar (adjust to taste)

- 1/2 lime, cut into wedges

- 2 ounces white rum

- 1 cup ice cubes

- Club soda

- Mango slices for garnish (optional)

Instructions:

1. **Muddle the Mango and Mint:**

   - In a cocktail shaker or a glass, muddle the fresh mango chunks and mint leaves together. Muddling helps release the flavors from the mint and mango.

2. **Add Sugar and Lime:**

   - Add sugar to the mango and mint mixture. Squeeze the lime wedges into the mixture, making sure to extract the juice. Drop

the squeezed lime wedges into
the shaker as well.

3. **Add Rum and Ice:**

   - Pour the white rum over the
     muddled ingredients. Add the ice
     cubes to the shaker.

4. **Shake Well:**

   - Close the shaker and shake the
     mixture well for about 15-20
     seconds. This helps chill the
     ingredients and combine the
     flavors.

5. **Strain into a Glass:**

   - Strain the mixture into a glass
     filled with ice. You can use a fine
     mesh strainer to remove the
     pulp if you prefer a smoother
     drink.

6. **Top with Club Soda:**

   - Top the drink with club soda for
     a fizzy finish. You can adjust the
     amount of club soda based on

your preference for the level of
carbonation.

7. **Garnish:**

- Garnish the Mango Mojito with
  a sprig of mint and, if desired, a
  slice of fresh mango on the rim
  of the glass.

8. **Serve:**

- Give the drink a gentle stir with
  a straw or a spoon before
  serving.

Mango Breakfast Delights

Mango Pancakes

Mango pancakes are a delicious and fruity twist on traditional pancakes. Here's a simple recipe for you to try:

Ingredients:

- 1 cup all-purpose flour
- 2 tablespoons sugar
- 1 teaspoon baking powder
- 1/2 teaspoon baking soda
- 1/4 teaspoon salt
- 3/4 cup buttermilk
- 1 large egg
- 2 tablespoons melted butter
- 1 teaspoon vanilla extract
- 1 ripe mango, peeled, pitted, and diced

Instructions:

1. **Mix Dry Ingredients:** In a large bowl, whisk together the flour, sugar, baking powder, baking soda, and salt.

2. **Mix Wet Ingredients:** In another bowl, whisk together the buttermilk, egg, melted butter, and vanilla extract.

3. **Combine Wet and Dry Ingredients:** Pour the wet ingredients into the dry ingredients and stir until just combined. Be careful not to overmix; a few lumps are okay.

4. **Add Mango:** Gently fold in the diced mango into the pancake batter.

5. **Preheat Griddle or Pan:** Preheat a griddle or non-stick pan over medium heat. Lightly grease it with butter or cooking spray.

6. **Cook Pancakes:** Pour 1/4 cup of batter onto the griddle for each pancake. Cook until bubbles form on the surface, then flip and cook until the other side is golden brown.

7. **Serve:** Once cooked, transfer the pancakes to a plate. You can serve

them with additional mango slices, a drizzle of maple syrup, or a dollop of whipped cream.

8. **Enjoy:** Serve the mango pancakes warm and enjoy the delicious combination of fluffy pancakes and sweet mango.

Mango Yogurt Parfait

A Mango Yogurt Parfait is a delicious and refreshing layered dessert or breakfast option that combines the sweetness of ripe mangoes with the creamy goodness of yogurt. Here's a simple recipe for you:

Ingredients:

1. Ripe mangoes, peeled, pitted, and diced

2. Greek yogurt or your favorite yogurt

3. Granola (store-bought or homemade)

4. Honey or maple syrup (optional, for added sweetness)

5. Fresh mint leaves for garnish (optional)

Instructions:

1. **Prepare the Mangoes:**

    - Peel the mangoes and cut them into small, bite-sized cubes. You can also puree some of the mango for a smoother texture if desired.

2. **Assemble the Parfait:**

    - In serving glasses or bowls, start by adding a layer of yogurt at the bottom.

    - Add a layer of diced mangoes on top of the yogurt.

    - Sprinkle a layer of granola over the mangoes. This adds a delightful crunch to the parfait.

    - Repeat the layers until you reach the top of the glass, finishing with a layer of granola and a few pieces of diced mango on top.

3. **Drizzle with Honey (Optional):**

- If you like your parfait a bit sweeter, drizzle honey or maple syrup over the top.

4. **Garnish (Optional):**

   - Garnish the parfait with fresh mint leaves for a burst of color and additional freshness.

5. **Serve Immediately:**

   - Serve the mango yogurt parfait immediately to enjoy the contrast of textures and flavors.

6. **Variations:**

   - Feel free to customize your parfait by adding other fruits like berries or sliced bananas.

   - Experiment with different types of yogurt, such as vanilla or coconut-flavored yogurt, to add more variety to the taste.

Mango Oatmeal Smoothie Bowl

Certainly! A Mango Oatmeal Smoothie Bowl is a delicious and nutritious way to start your day. Here's a simple recipe for you:

Ingredients:

- 1 cup frozen mango chunks
- 1/2 cup rolled oats
- 1/2 cup Greek yogurt (or any yogurt of your choice)
- 1/2 cup milk (dairy or plant-based)
- 1 tablespoon honey or maple syrup (optional, depending on your sweetness preference)
- Toppings of your choice (e.g., sliced banana, chia seeds, shredded coconut, nuts, granola)

Instructions:

1. **Blend the Smoothie:**
    - In a blender, combine the frozen mango chunks, rolled oats,

Greek yogurt, milk, and honey
or maple syrup.

- Blend until smooth and creamy. If the consistency is too thick, you can add more milk to reach your desired thickness.

2. **Assemble the Bowl:**

- Pour the smoothie into a bowl.

3. **Add Toppings:**

- Top your smoothie bowl with your favorite toppings. Sliced banana, chia seeds, shredded coconut, nuts, and granola are all great choices.

4. **Serve and Enjoy:**

- Grab a spoon and enjoy your delicious Mango Oatmeal Smoothie Bowl!

Feel free to customize the recipe to suit your taste preferences. You can also experiment with different toppings and add-ins like protein powder, flaxseeds, or a handful of spinach for an extra nutritional boost.

Mango Snacks for Movie Nights

Baked Mango Chip

Baked mango chips are a delicious and healthy snack that you can easily make at home. Here's a simple recipe for baked mango chips:

Ingredients:

- 2 ripe mangoes

- 1 tablespoon lemon juice (optional, to prevent browning)

- 1-2 teaspoons chili powder (optional, for a spicy kick)

- 1-2 teaspoons sugar (optional, depending on your preference)

Instructions:

1. **Preheat your oven:** Preheat your oven to 200°F (93°C). Line a baking sheet

with parchment paper or use a silicone baking mat.

2. **Prepare the mangoes:** Peel the mangoes and slice them thinly. The thinner the slices, the crispier the chips will be. You can use a mandoline slicer for even and thin slices.

3. **Optional lemon juice:** If you want to prevent the mango slices from browning, toss them in a bowl with lemon juice.

4. **Seasoning (optional):** In a separate bowl, mix together chili powder and sugar. Adjust the quantities to suit your taste. Toss the mango slices in this mixture until they are evenly coated.

5. **Arrange on the baking sheet:** Place the mango slices on the prepared baking sheet in a single layer. Make sure they are not touching each other to allow for even baking.

6. **Bake:** Bake in the preheated oven for 2-3 hours, or until the mango chips are dry and crispy. The time may vary depending on the thickness of your

slices and your oven, so keep an eye on them.

7. **Cool:** Once the mango chips are done, remove them from the oven and let them cool completely on the baking sheet. They will continue to crisp up as they cool.

8. **Store:** Store the baked mango chips in an airtight container at room temperature. Enjoy them as a healthy snack!

Mango Salsa Nachos

Mango salsa nachos are a delightful and refreshing twist on traditional nachos, incorporating the sweet and tangy flavors of mango salsa to complement the savory and cheesy elements. Here's a simple recipe for mango salsa nachos:

Ingredients:

For Mango Salsa:

- 1 large ripe mango, diced

- 1/2 red onion, finely chopped

- 1 red bell pepper, diced

- 1/4 cup fresh cilantro, chopped

- 1 jalapeño, seeds removed and finely chopped

- Juice of 1 lime

- Salt and pepper to taste

For Nachos:

- Tortilla chips

- Shredded cheese (cheddar, Monterey Jack, or a blend)

- Black beans, drained and rinsed

- Sliced jalapeños (optional, for extra heat)

- Sour cream (optional, for serving)

- Guacamole (optional, for serving)

Instructions:

1. **Prepare the Mango Salsa:**

   - In a bowl, combine the diced mango, red onion, red bell

pepper, cilantro, jalapeño, and
lime juice.

- Season with salt and pepper to taste.

- Mix well and set aside to allow the flavors to meld.

2. **Assemble the Nachos:**

- Preheat your oven to 375°F (190°C).

- On a large baking sheet or oven-safe dish, arrange a layer of tortilla chips.

- Sprinkle a generous amount of shredded cheese over the chips.

- Add black beans evenly across the chips and cheese.

3. **Bake the Nachos:**

- Place the baking sheet or dish in the preheated oven and bake until the cheese is melted and bubbly, usually about 8-10 minutes.

4. **Add Mango Salsa:**

    - Once the nachos are out of the
      oven, spoon the prepared mango
      salsa over the melted cheese and
      beans.

5. **Optional Toppings:**

    - If desired, add sliced jalapeños
      for an extra kick.

    - Serve with dollops of sour cream
      and guacamole on the side.

6. **Serve Immediately:**

    - Mango salsa nachos are best
      enjoyed immediately while the
      chips are still crispy and the
      cheese is gooey.

These mango salsa nachos are a perfect
combination of sweet, savory, and spicy
flavors. Feel free to customize the recipe
based on your preferences, adding ingredients
like diced avocado or a squeeze of additional
lime juice.

Mango and Chili Popcorn

Mango and chili popcorn is a unique and flavorful twist on traditional popcorn. It combines the sweetness of ripe mango with the heat of chili to create a delicious and satisfying snack. Here's a simple recipe you can try at home:

Ingredients:

- Popcorn kernels

- Ripe mango (pureed or finely chopped)

- Chili powder or cayenne pepper (adjust to taste)

- Butter or oil for popping popcorn

- Salt to taste

Instructions:

1. **Pop the Popcorn:**

   - Pop the popcorn kernels using your preferred method, whether it's on the stovetop, using an air popper, or microwave popcorn.

2. **Prepare Mango Puree:**

- Peel and pit a ripe mango, then puree the flesh in a blender or food processor until smooth. Alternatively, finely chop the mango into small pieces.

3. **Season the Popcorn:**

   - In a large bowl, drizzle the popped popcorn with melted butter or oil, ensuring even coverage.

4. **Add Mango Flavor:**

   - Spoon the mango puree or chopped mango over the popcorn. Toss the popcorn to coat it evenly with the mango flavor. You can start with a small amount and add more to your liking.

5. **Spice it Up:**

   - Sprinkle chili powder or cayenne pepper over the popcorn. Start with a small amount and adjust according to your spice preference. The combination of sweet mango and spicy chili creates a delightful contrast.

6. **Toss and Mix:**

   - Toss the popcorn well to ensure that the mango and chili are evenly distributed. You can use a large spoon or your hands (make sure they are clean) to mix everything thoroughly.

7. **Adjust Seasoning:**

   - Taste a few pieces and adjust the seasoning as needed. You can add more mango puree, chili powder, or salt according to your taste preferences.

8. **Serve and Enjoy:**

   - Once you're satisfied with the flavor, serve the mango and chili popcorn immediately. It's best enjoyed fresh, but you can store any leftovers in an airtight container.

Tips and Tricks for Cooking with Mango

Cutting and Peeling Mangoes

It should go without saying that there are several approaches to peeling and slicing a mango. However, throughout the years I've experimented with several approaches of cutting mangoes, and I'm going to share with you the strategies that have consistently produced the greatest results for me.

When I attempted to cut into a mango for the first time, I had no idea that there was a huge pit hidden inside. But I had a very immediate realization of what was going on when I attempted to chop the mango exactly down the middle and my knife struck it!

Even at that point, I was completely unaware of the depth of the abyss. Then I shifted the position of my knife slightly and attempted chopping once again, but I kept hitting the pit...again...and again.

To begin, there are several types of mangoes. Even while the tastes of these different species may be distinct from one another, their "anatomy," if you will, is fundamentally the same.

BIG FAT MANGOES

I'm aware that comparing them to "big fat mangoes" isn't exactly scientific, but it's the analogy that comes to me whenever I think about them.

They may be referred to by a number of various names depending on where you are in the world; nevertheless, despite these variations, they are all extremely comparable. The skins of the large, plump mangoes exhibit a variety of colors, including green, red, and yellow. I'd guess that around twenty years ago, many of these types of mangoes had a higher fiber content, which made them somewhat more difficult to cut. However, in today's world, it is very uncommon to come across examples that are richer in meat, have a lower percentage of fibrous content, and maintain their shape when cut.

When you try to peel and cut these large mangoes, you may find that you have a difficult time doing so since they are rather cumbersome. Therefore, I begin by severing a portion of the base around the point where the stem was linked.

SMALL YELLOW MANGOES

Again, "small yellow mangoes" is not a particularly scientific categorization; but, in essence, these mangoes are smaller in size compared to the "big fat" mangoes, and their skin is immediately distinguishable due to the fact that it is brilliant yellow.

You may know them as Mexican Ataulfo, honey, or jade mangoes. Here in Hong Kong, we frequently receive Philippine mangoes, which are also known as Manila mangoes. You may also know them as jade mangoes or honey mangoes. They have a lower density than the larger ones, and their flavor and sweetness tend to be more concentrated.

Storing Mangoes Properly

Again, "small yellow mangoes" is not a particularly scientific categorization; but, in essence, these mangoes are smaller in size compared to the "big fat" mangoes, and their skin is immediately distinguishable due to the fact that it is brilliant yellow.

Mangoes from the Philippines are frequently available to us here in Hong Kong. The level of ripeness of the mangoes is a crucial factor in determining how they should be stored; you might have guessed this before. The refrigerator is not the ideal storage environment for unripe mangoes; rather, they should be kept at room temperature. Over the course of a few days, when left at room temperature, the fruits will continue to mature, becoming sweeter and more tender as the time passes. Place unripe mangoes in a paper bag at room temperature. This will hasten the process of ripening the mangoes. When the mango gives just a little bit in response to gentle pressure, it's ready to eat.

If your mango is already ripe, there is no need to wait any longer to enjoy it. much though they are wonderful on their own, ripe mangoes are much better when blended into your morning smoothie, used as a topping for oatmeal, or even chopped up and baked into a cake. All of these preparations result in a delectable flavor.mangoes that are often referred to as honey mangoes, jade mangoes, or Mexican Ataulfo mangoes are another name for these fruits. They have a lower density than the larger ones, and their flavor and sweetness tend to be more concentrated.

Can You Store Mangoes in the Fridge?

Mangoes are perfectly suited to being kept in the refrigerator for extended periods of time. Put it in the refrigerator if you have a ripe mango but aren't quite ready to eat it yet. In fact, you should do that if you find yourself with a ripe mango but aren't quite ready to eat it. You will have a little bit more time to appreciate the fruit since the ripening process will be slowed down by the chilly temperature that is found inside the refrigerator. Mangoes that are ripe and whole can be stored in the

refrigerator for approximately five days
without losing their freshness.

Can You Freeze Mangoes?

Yes, you can absolutely freeze mangoes. In
fact, they are one of the fruits that freeze
exceptionally well. To properly freeze a
mango, wait until it's ripe and then follow the
steps below:

1. Peel the ripe mango and cut it into
    slices or cubes.

2. Arrange the mango pieces on a baking
    sheet lined with parchment paper,
    making sure that none of the pieces
    touch each other.

3. Place the baking sheet in the freezer for
    at least two hours, up to overnight.

4. Once the fruit pieces are frozen,
    transfer them to a freezer-safe bag and
    squeeze as much air out of the bag as
    possible. Seal the bag tightly and label it
    with the date.

Mango will maintain its flavor for as long as six months after being frozen using this technique. Putting frozen mango in the refrigerator for the night will allow it to thaw, or you may throw the bags of frozen mango pieces in a kettle of cold water to speed up the process. In around three hours, the fruit should have defrosted completely.

Substituting Mango in Recipes

1. Peach

Peaches are supposed to have originated in China thousands of years before mangoes, making them close relatives of the tropical fruit. This fruit's exterior is fuzzy, and its meat can be either white or yellow.

Peaches have a naturally sweet flavor, and peaches cooked in syrup take the cake for flavor and popularity, but they pack a hefty calorie punch. The peach already has quite a considerable quantity of sugars (about 33 g per fruit), making it one of those fruits you want to consume with caution; yet, it is a nutritious snack, especially after physical exercise. Peaches can be found in the stone fruit family.

This fruit is frequently regarded as the most suitable alternative to mango, and it also functions well when used to flavor mixed drinks in place of mango nectar.

Peaches have their own unique flavor, so they won't taste the same as mangoes, but the consistency and color of peaches are quite similar to that of mangoes, and this makes them a suitable substitute for mango in any recipe that calls for it.

Nectarine

The ancestry of the peach cultivar known as nectarines is unknown. Others contend that it was originally developed in China about the same time as peaches and was brought to the United States by the Spanish. The former theory holds that it was bred in California in the 1940s in an effort to achieve a peach variety that had a more earthy flavor.

With the exception of their rinds, the two fruits are virtually indistinguishable from one another. Nectarines, on the other hand, do not have the characteristically fuzzy skin that peaches possess.

Because of this, nectarines are a wonderful alternative for peaches in cooked meals. This is due to the fact that the skin of peaches becomes excessively tough when they are cooked, but the skin of nectarines is significantly thinner and does not need to be peeled before they are cooked.

Nectarines are an excellent source of several essential minerals, including potassium, folate, antioxidants, phosphorus, beta-carotene, as well as vitamins A, K, and C. In addition, nectarines are an excellent source of hydration due to the fact that they are composed of 85 percent water (per 100 grams).

Smoothies, fruit salads, and baked goods may all benefit greatly from the addition of this fruit as a mango substitute.

Conclusion

It is a beautiful voyage that not only titillates the taste senses but also develops a sense of togetherness and joy around the dinner table. Exploring mango dishes for the whole family is a wonderful way to spend time together as a family. Because of their adaptability, mangoes may be used in a broad variety of recipes, ranging from energizing smoothies to savory salads and indulgent desserts. As a result, it is simple to accommodate the many tastes that may exist within a family. These mango dishes bring a blast of flavor as well as a healthy dose of nutrients to your meals, and they are perfect for enjoying on a warm day or as a sweet finish to a meal with the family. By embracing the richness of this tropical fruit, one not only delights their taste buds but also builds memories that will last a lifetime, transforming regular dinners for the entire family into spectacular occasions. So go ahead and indulge in the succulent flavor of mangoes, and let the time spent together enjoying a delectable dish to draw you and the people you care about even closer.

www.ingramcontent.com/pod-product-compliance
Lightning Source LLC
Chambersburg PA
CBHW070850260726

48661CB00004B/1331